ALISON DAVIES

Illustrated by Alexandra Kern

sleep
tight

ILLUSTRATED BEDTIME STORIES &
MEDITATIONS TO SOOTHE YOU TO SLEEP

First published in the UK in 2021 by
Leaping Hare Press
An imprint of The Quarto Group
The Old Brewery, 6 Blundell Street
London N7 9BH, United Kingdom
T (0)20 7700 6700 F (0)20 7700 8066
www.QuartoKnows.com

British Library Cataloguing-in-Publication Data
A catalogue record for this book is available from the British Library

ISBN: 978-0-7112-6181-5

This book was conceived, designed and produced by
Leaping Hare Press
58 West Street, Brighton BN1 2RA, United Kingdom
Publisher Richard Green
Art Director Paileen Currie
Editorial Director Jennifer Barr
Commissioning Editor Chloe Murphy
Designer Nikki Ellis

Printed in China

10 9 8 7 6 5 4 3 2 1

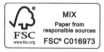

Contents

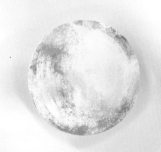

Introduction

THE POWER OF STORYTELLING

Since the dawn of humanity stories have captivated us, transporting us to new places. From those first tentative steps of our early ancestors into a bright new world, as the challenges of the day were faced and then later shared around the campfire in tales of those exploits, stories are a part of the web of life. Each delicate strand builds a common landscape that helps connect us to each other. In those early days, narratives were concocted to make sense of the world, to explain what must have seemed like a supernatural phenomenon, something that only the gods could have created. From the rising sun to sky-splitting flashes of lightning, Mother Nature has always been the best storyteller. The changing of the seasons prompted great tales, epic sagas that would stand the test of time. And while the oral tradition flourished, so too did our understanding of words and our ability to create pictures through the tales we told so fluently.

Narratives come in all shapes and sizes but the one thing they have in common is their ability to bring us together. Stories help strangers to bond, friends to smile and loved ones to remember treasured moments. They are great learning tools. A concept slipped between the pages of your favourite book will stay with you forever. When you hear or read a story, your mind relaxes, allowing you to take it in. As the words wrap around you and combine with images to conjure emotion, the message in the narrative soaks deep beneath your skin. Once a story has become a part of you, all you have to do is bring it to mind to re-experience that feeling.

STORIES AS A TOOL FOR SELF-CARE

Stories have been with you since the day you were born, and while you might have your favourites from childhood, the tales you tell yourself are the most powerful. The constant chatter inside your head is an ongoing narrative that affects the way you think and feel. Change this narrative and you will change your life.

You can use the power of storytelling for spiritual self-care and to transform your outlook each day. Using a powerful guided meditation which puts you at the centre of the tale as part of your night-time ritual is an effective practice for wellbeing. You'll feel more relaxed as the narrative switches your focus from the stresses of the day, and the story will remain in your subconscious, where it will reprogram your thoughts and actions.

HOW TO USE THIS BOOK

This book is a compendium of guided bedtime meditations. Each one will calm you and ease you into a particular mindset. Want to feel inspired and get your creative mojo back? Do you need to find clarity or conjure inner strength to face the challenges of the day ahead? Before you go to sleep each night, find the right meditation for you in this book and read it with passion.

Visualize yourself inside the meditation and play it back in your mind like a film until you fall asleep. Use your imagination to conjure the tale, allow it to guide you into sleep, and then let your subconscious do the rest.

When you wake up, read the affirmations included at the end of the meditation and repeat them to yourself throughout the day. If you need an extra boost, I've included a practical exercise at the end of each meditation to help you maintain your good mindset.

From building confidence to seeking and finding patience, it's all possible. Each narrative holds the secret and will help you move closer to your goal. Take your time and allow the storyline to unfold. Engage your senses and let the tale work its magic in your soul. Become like a child again, open and ready for enchantment. Before you know it, nothing will be able to hold you back, and you'll be on a journey to the moon.

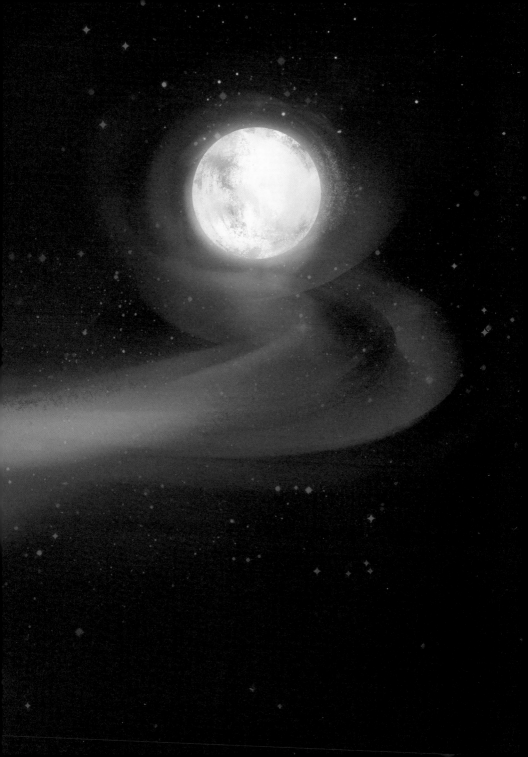

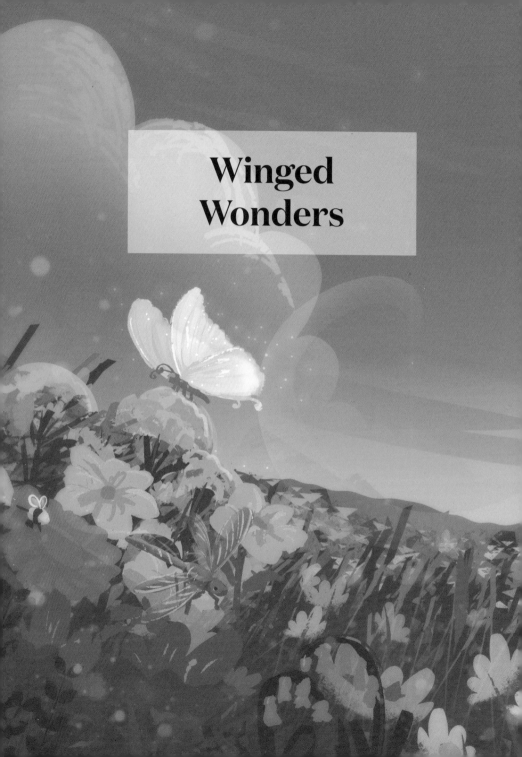

Winged
Wonders

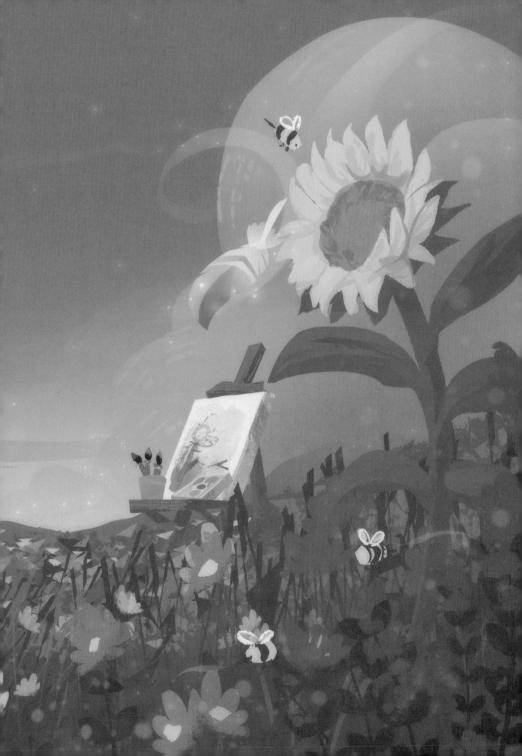

A GUIDED NARRATIVE TO:

Promote creativity

—

Stretch the imagination

You are standing in a field of wildflowers, beautiful gems all the colours of the rainbow. It's the height of summer but there's a hint of a breeze, enough to make the tiny blooms bend and weave. They look like dancing fireflies. The air is sweet, and you draw in a deep invigorating breath, taking it into your lungs. You are buzzing with energy, so much so that you begin to run, skipping through the undergrowth in no particular direction. You imagine you're a feather caught in the wind. Around and around you spin, arms outstretched.

A bee hums its melody in your ear and you're suddenly aware of all the winged insects flitting and hovering, jumping from flower to flower. Butterflies with delicate gossamer wings and huge eye-shaped patterns dance before you. Dragonflies with their metallic wings join in the parade, swapping partners and directions with the flick of a tail. A turquoise damselfly circles you, a darting ribbon of light leading you in a pirouette. All the creatures of the earth, of Mother Nature, have come to perform for you. Suddenly you want to join in with their capers and be a part of the show, to create something out of nothing, like these winged wonders on display. But what talents do you have and where to start?

As if in answer to your question, a translucent butterfly lands in the palm of your hand. Its wings are deeply veined and the colour of pearl. As you look again, you notice that it's changing form, transforming before your eyes. The wings are gone, the body is solid and lengthy, and you realize you are now holding a paintbrush. Your palm tingles with excitement. This is your chance to create something new. To paint your own portrait and make it real. Your fingers twitch and soon you are working away, using the air in front of you as your easel and canvas. *You see with your imagination.* There's no thought behind it, you let your innate creativity take over. Your wrist flicks as you splash swirls of light with an invisible palette. A pattern emerges, a carnival of colour and movement as the painting takes shape in your mind. Only you know what it is, the subject is of your choosing. Around you, the winged wonders gather to watch. They know something special is about to happen.

When you are ready, you take a step back. Pause to survey your masterpiece. It is a work of art because it comes from your soul. It captures the very essence of who you are. Inside you feel a flicker of warmth. *The creative spark has been ignited.*

The picture becomes a reality, not just a figment of your imagination, but flesh and blood. Framed and catching the sunlight it stands upon the grass and you marvel at your creation. The more you gaze at it, the bigger it becomes. Growing and spreading until it is no longer a portrait, but a portal the size of a window. Instinctively you step through, into your picture. You find yourself in a world of your own making. Everything feels comfortable here. There is nothing to fear because you know this place inside out. This is the seat of your imagination, the place where all things start.

You smile and say, '*I am a creative being!*'

Behind you is a giant waterfall, it cascades down into a deep ravine where each droplet of water meets and becomes something new, just as your thoughts form ideas in your mind. With every step you take you feel more energized. You know that you can be anything you want, because you are the artist, the inventor, the force behind everything. Your reality is a result of all the choices you have made up until this moment. Which means that *every choice and action that follows creates a new destiny*.

Nothing is impossible.

When you are ready you take a step back through the portal, through the picture and into your reality, but you are not alone. You bring inspiration and a renewed verve for life with you. *Your imagination is on fire*. The meadow greets you like an old friend, and you feel lucky to be alive. The sun is slipping from its place in the sky and everything is bathed in an amber glow. The subtle changes bring a different kind of beauty to the landscape and you realize that each moment has something new to offer. *There is potential in every second*.

Time may be ebbing, bringing this day to a close, but there is always another one waiting on the brow of the hill. A chance to start the story again, to let your creativity flow and express who you are. As night falls and you settle under the veil of stars, you feel at peace. *You are ready to unleash your imagination and make your mark on the world.*

Affirmations

———

'I ignite my creative spark.'

'There is potential in every moment.'

'I see with my imagination.'

'Every day is an opportunity to express myself.'

Boost your mindset

Use this creative exercise to switch up your thinking!

Pick something routine that you do every day, for example walking the dog, making a cup of tea, checking your emails. Write a couple of sentences about this.

Now imagine that what you have in front of you is the outline for the next big blockbuster movie. It's up to you to come up with an exciting billboard poster with a caption to sell this. For example, on making a brew you might say 'It was an ordinary day, an ordinary girl, but a steamy encounter was about to change everything!' Be creative and let your mind wander. You can draw your ideas or create the vision in your head.

When you spend a few minutes thinking creatively about everyday scenarios your perspective shifts. You see the wonder in the world and flex your imagination. It also puts you in a positive frame of mind.

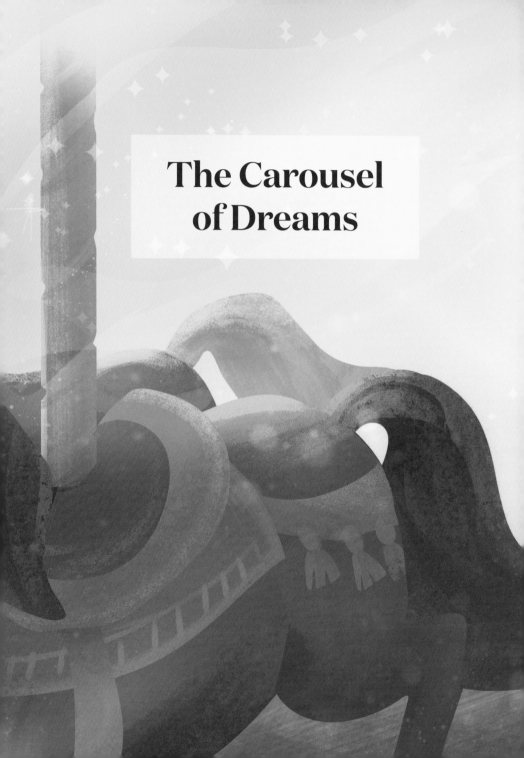

The Carousel of Dreams

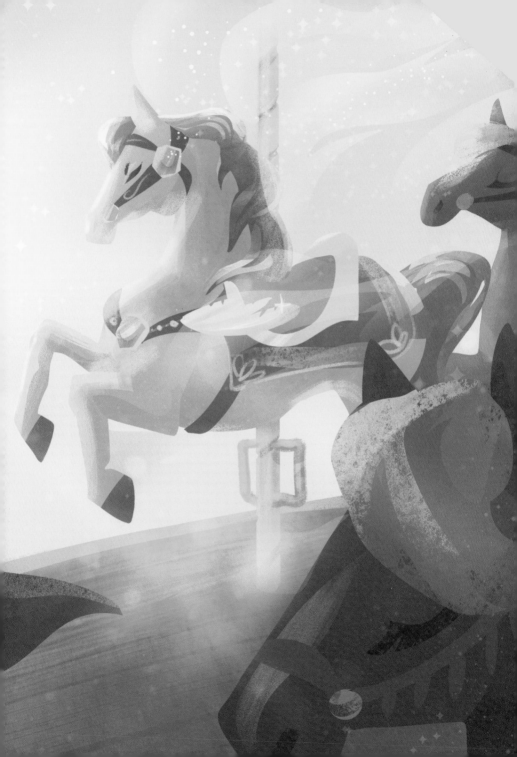

Unleash joy

—

Create an attitude of wonder

The bright colours of the carousel are the first thing to catch your eye. Glittering golds, sunshine yellows, rich crimson and sky blue, mixed in a whirl of pattern. They daub the characters, the chariots and the horses that move in a slow, rhythmic waltz. Then comes the music; the chime of pretty bells, a cheerful melody that lifts your heart. You can't help but smile. It reminds you of childhood, of family days out, celebrations and fun. All the treats of the fair are captured in this one ride, and suddenly you can't think of anything better than clambering on board in the hope that you'll steal some of that youthful energy for yourself.

The white horse with the golden mane and bridle is your steed. You fit snugly in the saddle, just in time for the ride to begin. The music fires up, an anthem of joy. The carousel spins, slow and steady. There is no race, only the pleasure of the moment. A gentle breeze caresses your face and you close your eyes. The circular movement of the ride reminds you that life is a continual cycle.

Your head drops. Your chest loosens.
Your jaw slackens.

You take a deep breath and feel yourself physically relax. The cloak of stress that you have been carrying slips easily from your shoulders and *you feel instantly lighter and brighter*.

Something shifts beneath you and without opening your eyes, you know that something has changed. Enchantment is everywhere, and you realize that you are no longer part of the carousel. That you have lifted into the air, upon the back of this magical horse with wings. Its golden mane is cool against your fingers, white sinewy muscles flex, and wings stretch out from taut shoulder blades. Your spirit soars as the steed lifts higher. The feeling of freedom, of rapture and release takes over and you let out a cry of delight, howling into the wind.

Bliss is this moment, this feeling, right now.

The fluffy white clouds gather at your feet, as your steed dips and swoops. You can see everything from up here. Thick plateaus of green, like a patchwork of fields. The tips of mountains, and the darker green clusters of forest. The sun spills down and the warmth caresses you. The sky, your backdrop, seems to change colour, going from burnt orange to a soft peach and then a deep rose pink. *The colours soothe your soul and you feel a wave of contentment wash over you.*

Happy memories of the people and the places that always make you smile come to mind now. You touch a hand to your heart as you think of these things, and when you pull it away you find a piece of rose quartz nestled in your palm. All the joy of this moment, all of the love that you are feeling is captured in this beautiful stone. You hold the soft pink crystal against your cheek and feel the energy seep beneath your skin.

And you realize then that you're not just talking about this uplifting experience, as much as you are thankful for it, *you are also grateful for all of the blessings in your life*. You think then of the good things, big and small, that grace your world. Little things, like that first morning coffee, or your favourite song on the radio. Beautiful moments that will stay with you, like a gorgeous sunset with the one you love and the sound of birdsong on a spring morning. *There are so many things to be grateful for, and that makes you truly happy.*

As the sky once more changes colour, darkening with the coming of evening, you return to earth. The carousel turns, and you step lightly from your perch, feet skimming the ground. The earth welcomes you and everything is normal. Except that when you look around now, everything seems to shimmer with stardust, as if touched by magic, and you realize there's wonder to be found in each moment. *Happiness is yours for the taking.* It's a choice, a thankful feeling that everything is as it should be in your life. Pulling the rose quartz from your pocket, you smile, and it spreads from your heart to every part of your being.

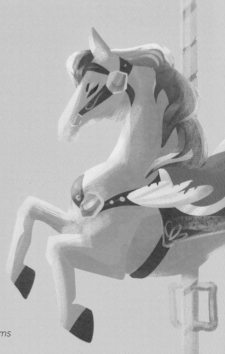

Affirmations

—

'I choose happiness.'

'Bliss is in this moment, right now.'

'I see the wonder in my world.'

'I am blessed.'

Boost your mindset

Shift your perspective and see the joy in your life with this exercise!

Invest in a keepsake box and fill it with good memories, anything from photographs to mementos of days out, tickets, pictures, happy quotes, and poems etc. You can also write up special memories as short stories and include these in the box.

Every evening, spend some time thinking about the day and all the things you are thankful for. These could be little things, like a nice home-cooked meal or a friendly smile from a stranger, to bigger events. Remember to also give thanks for all the things that make you special, and for family and friends too. Write a list of these blessings on some paper and add this to your keepsake box. At the end of each week, or whenever you need a pick-me-up, dip into the box and draw something out to remind you of the joy that's present in every day.

Get into the habit of being grateful and you'll see the blessings in life more easily. You will also switch your focus from the things you feel are lacking, to all the good things you have. This promotes a positive attitude and re-enforces a sense of wellbeing.

The Lake
of Tranquillity

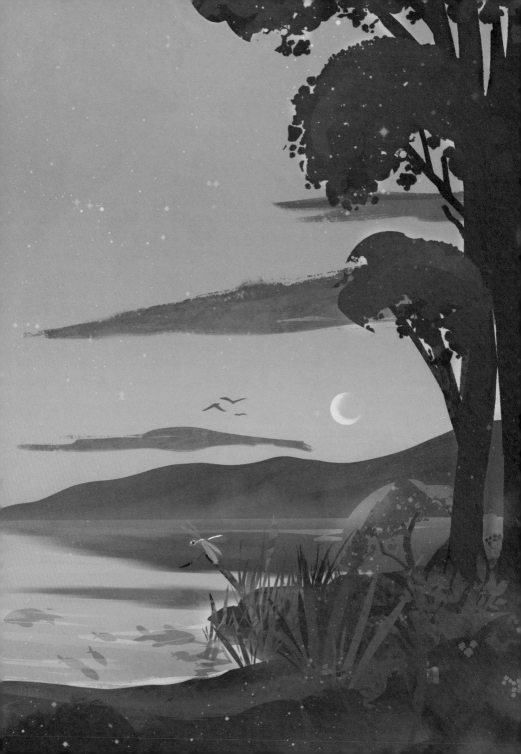

A GUIDED NARRATIVE TO:

Promote inner peace

—

Feel calm and connected

It is first light, and you are standing before an enormous lake. The sun peeps over the horizon, its gentle rays dance upon the surface of the water.
It is as if you are looking at a giant mural, a wall of serenity. The air is fresh but warm against your skin. In the distance you see birds, flitting from perches in the trees and hedgerows. They are just waking up, like you. The landscape before you is muted, soft greens merge with the powder blue slick of the sky, the water is a silver river at your feet, and you can't help but wonder what delights lie beneath. If you took a peek, would you find an underwater world buzzing with activity or would there be nothing but liquid stillness?

A sapphire dragonfly skims the water's edge, scouting the area for movement. It catches your eye, and you follow its dance as it circuits the pond. Nothing else matters at this moment. You are entranced, all of your attention on the scene before you. Calm permeates every pore of your being, and you let out a deep sigh.

'*Be still.*'

'*Be calm.*'

'*Be pure.*'

'*Just be.*'

The mantra slips easily into your mind, and it fits with how you feel right now. A spiral of light captures your attention. It glistens beneath the water, and you realize that it's the sun's reflection as it gets higher in the sky. As you watch, you notice outward ripples travelling in small circles, as if something is stirring beneath. Warmed by the heat of the sun, the lake is coming to life. And you feel it too, like a flower opening in your heart, *you feel awake and at peace with the world.*

You are composed and ready for what lies ahead.

You step towards the sloping bank, your feet tripping lightly towards the water's edge. Bending forwards, you dip in a hand and feel the cool acceptance of the lake drawing you closer. It's inviting you in, and you know you must accept. You long to submerge every part of your body, to be enclosed in this peaceful realm.

Gradually you drift towards the centre of the pond, where the sparkling orb of the sun waits. The comforting warmth of the water slides over your shoulders, down your spine; it cushions your limbs. Again, you hear it, the voice in your head.

'Be still.'

'Be calm.'

'Just be.'

Each part of the mantra sings to your soul. *It's a reminder that you will always be able to find the silence within, that there's stillness in every moment if you take the time to look for it.*

You tread water on the spot. Your chin rests upon the surface and you breathe deeply. The surrounding vegetation rustles in the breeze. The sun, now fully in the sky, bathes everything in a golden glow and the colours that were once subdued now unleash their shine. Taking a deep breath, you dive underneath, aiming for the bed of the lake. As you swim, you see the fish slowly stirring. Their heads reaching up towards you, curious as to your presence but comfortable that you are in their world.

Iridescent scales dazzle your eyes and you are overcome with the beauty of this place. Quietness fills your mind, it swells until it swallows every worry and stressful thought that you have ever had.

'Be still.'

'Be calm.'

'Just be.'

You feel the words and know the sentiments behind each part of the mantra and what they mean for you. Like a magical charm, you don't need to speak or hear them; they are a part of you now.

The deep blue of the water is a satin sheet to your skin. It covers you delicately and *you feel sleepy, relaxed, completely content*. This is your sacred space where you will always find inner peace. Slowly you float towards the surface, as light as a feather. The sun's rays reach down for you, easing you upwards until you emerge in the centre of the pond. Still floating upon your back, your legs and arms stretched out like a human star, you smile. The silence of the underwater world remains in your heart, but you are greeted with new sounds now. A frog ribbits in the distance. A songbird tweets its pretty melody, and the water laps at the grassy bank. Nature is ready for a new day, and you are ready for anything because you hold the key to tranquillity in your heart.

Affirmations

———

'Serenity lives within me.'

'There is stillness in every moment.'

'The key to tranquillity is in my heart.'

'Be still, be calm, be pure, just be.'

Boost your mindset

Find an inner well of peace with this exercise, which uses the mantra from the story to instil serenity throughout the day.

Start by putting a stop to internal chatter. Every time a negative thought or criticism arises in your mind say 'Stop!' out loud or in your head.

Next, turn your attention to the way you are breathing. Slow down the rhythm by counting to four slowly as you breathe in and out, then extend each breath by one count. Repeat this cycle several times until you feel more relaxed.

When you are ready say the mantra, either in your head or out loud if circumstance allows. 'Be still, be calm, be pure, just be.' Think about each part of the mantra and what it means as you say it. Repeat several times, or until you feel calm.

The mantra switches the focus of the mind, taking you away from stressful thought patterns. The gentle repetitive rhythm combined with slow, deep breathing relaxes body and mind.

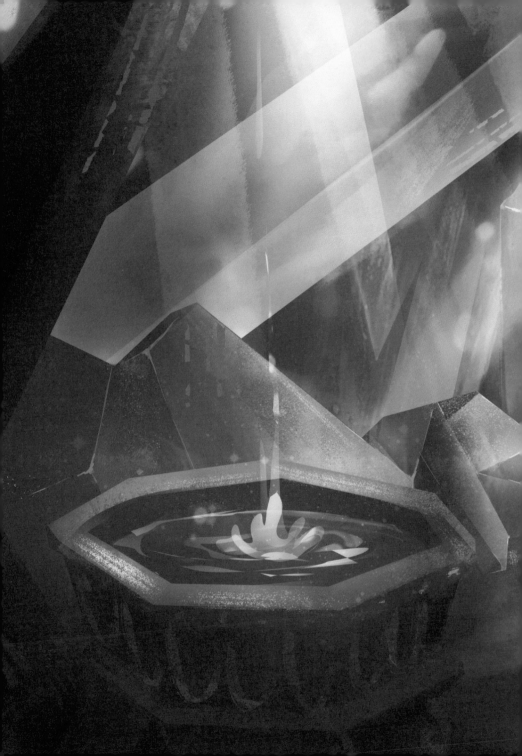

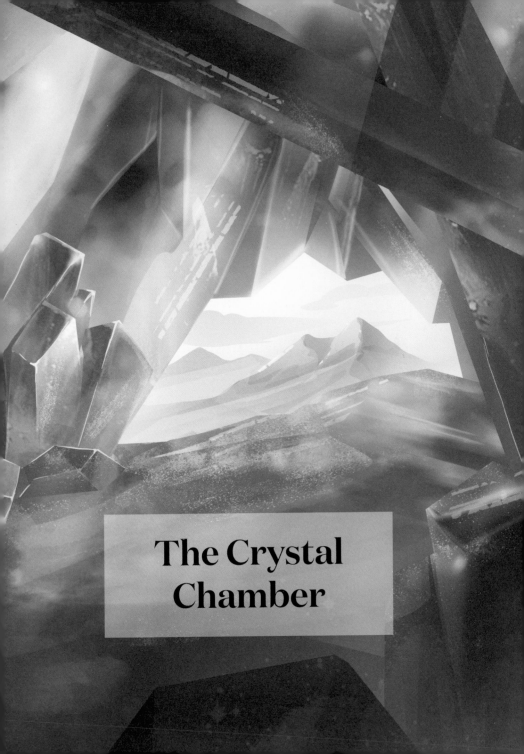

The Crystal Chamber

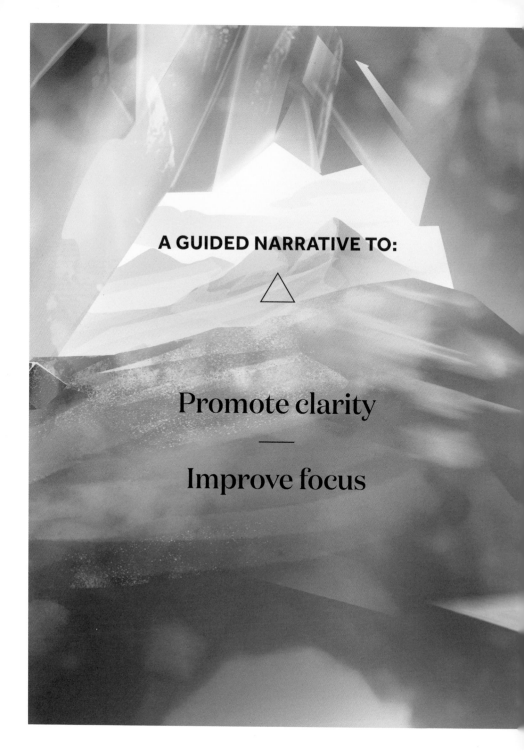

A GUIDED NARRATIVE TO:

Promote clarity

—

Improve focus

You stand on snow, feet sinking into the cold as a blizzard swirls around you. In the distance there are ice-capped mountains, their frosted peaks like pointed fingers poking the sky, but you cannot make out what's below them. The view is obscured, swathed in darkness. A mist gathers around your shoulders, and the curling tendrils of shadow beckon you closer. There's a ghost of a thought at the back of your mind, a realization that it's only by submerging yourself in the mire that you will finally emerge. You step deeper into the fog, wondering how you'll be able to see where you are going. You needn't worry, each step brings you further into the light until eventually *you see everything.*

Before you stands a yawning cavern made of quartz crystal like a giant ice palace; it takes your breath away. Rising into the clouds, the many facetted surface glimmers as a shaft of winter sunlight hits, and you are showered in sparkles. You peer inside, but there is only darkness, nothing to reveal what secrets lurk within this mammoth chamber. A question forms in your mind. What if you were to enter, what would you discover? The thought thrills you. It feels like you were meant to find this place. The wind wraps around you and with a final nudge you're inside, curiosity drawing you to the heart of the crystal.

Instantly, the darkness is replaced by diamond brightness. At every turn there are windows, all shapes and sizes, positioned from floor to ceiling and each one a chasm of light. You shield your eyes for a moment, letting them adjust to the change in environment. It's as if you've stepped into another world, a glittering realm where everything is crystal clear. There is no room for shadows, for half-formed ideas or muddy waters. *This is a place of complete clarity.*

You circle the chamber and notice an ornate plinth in the far corner, with a font in the centre. The water inside is rich, inky and purple, the colour of the deepest amethyst. You can't resist. You have to dip your hand in, to feel the pigment against your skin. The thick liquid caresses your fingers. The coolness slows your pulse and you feel comfortable. With a swishing motion you move the liquid, making patterns and shapes with your fingers. You begin to think of your life, of day-to-day dealings, letting any issues or problems rise to the surface, but instead of worrying you feel no attachment to these things. It's as if you have been removed from the situation. It still exists, but it does not affect you. You feel no emotion, no stress.

You are an objective observer, able to see with clear vision.

The water in the font ripples as you pull your hand away. It continues to move, swirls of colour fading to indigo then rose pink. Soon it is turning creamy white and then finally the sheer translucence of a freshwater stream. Your mind feels the same; no longer clogged with unnecessary thoughts, it is an airy room ready to home a new approach. All stress is gone, evaporated in a single breath and like the water, *your head is clear*.

You peer into the font again and this time notice pictures forming upon the surface. Images that you can relate to. It's as if the fluid within is a physical reflection of your inner state. Instantly you know what you must do. The direction that you must go in. You can see the way forwards and have a vision for the future. Any concerns or doubts slip away like dust and you feel certain of your path. Motivated by this fresh insight, you return to the cavern entrance, eager to get back to your world and put things in motion.

'Everything is crystal clear,' you say. The chamber rings at the sound of your voice and you marvel one last time at the magnificence of this magical place.

It is night as you leave the cavern. The sky is peppered with stars, and the snow feels smooth underfoot. It may be icy cold compared to the inner sanctum of the chamber, but you do not feel the chill.

You are focused.

An arrow seeking its target.

Negative thoughts may come and go, but they have no power over you, for you have the crystal chamber as your refuge. It is there within you, a safe space where *all becomes clear*. Knowing this simple fact, you can return home, to the comfort of your bed, and drift into dream.

Clarity is yours from this moment on and forever after.

Affirmations

___

'Everything is crystal clear.'

'I am an arrow, primed and ready to hit my target.'

'I see, I think, I am.'

'Clarity is mine from this moment in time.'

Boost your mindset

Invest in a quartz crystal to help you maintain clarity and focus.

Spend five minutes every day holding it in both hands. As you breathe in, imagine drawing the sparkling energy of the crystal inside you. To boost the positive effect, picture yourself cocooned in the crystal chamber. As you breathe out, pour any fear or confusion into the crystal.

At least once a week, take the crystal outside and bury it in the soil so that any negative energy can be absorbed by the earth and transformed into light. If you don't have access to a garden, then simply bury the crystal in a plant pot overnight or leave in a glass of salt water.

Once cleansed, you can pop the crystal beneath your pillow at night and ask for guidance in your dreams.

Quartz crystal amplifies and also transmits energy, making it the perfect stone to work with when you want to release negative energy and clear the mind. Breathing with the crystal helps to calm and focus the mind.

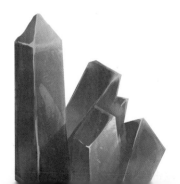

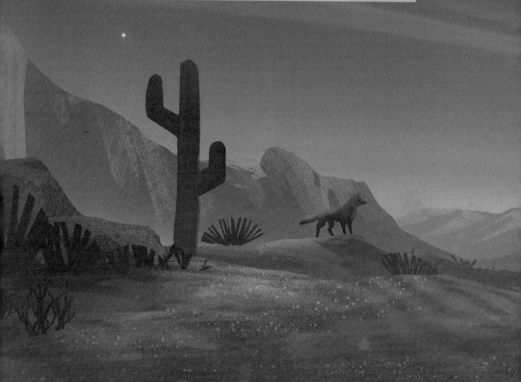

Desert
Dreamer

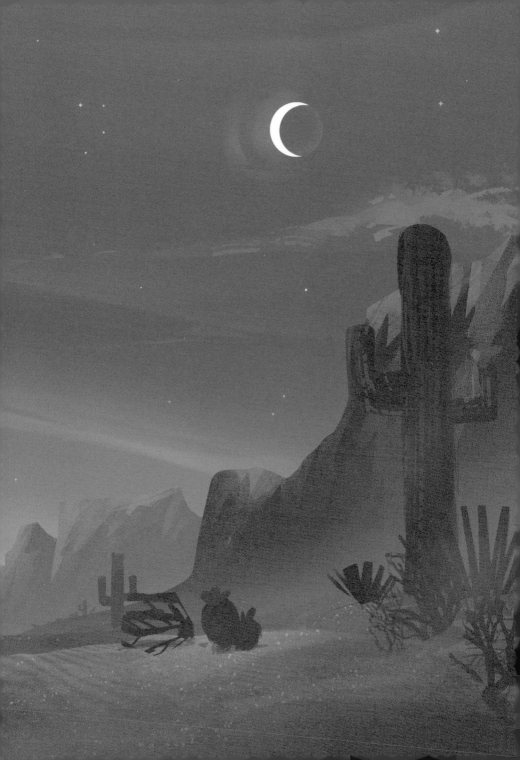

A GUIDED NARRATIVE TO:

Promote patience

—

Relinquish control and embrace the flow

You have been sleeping... resting... waiting.

You open your eyes, examine the vista, and find the landscape has changed. No soft cushioned bed with crisp white sheets, instead you find the dusty barren land is your mattress, the golden sun your blanket. The sky, a swirl of sea blue, glides above you. Every colour is fresh, vivid, breath-taking, as if it's just been painted by an artist. You take a moment to acclimatize and realize that the desert is your new home. You draw your hands over the baked earth, feel the thinly veined cracks against your skin. Something stirs inside, a longing, an old desire for something more, but at the same time you realize this is exactly where you need to be right now. *There is no pressure here, no need to strive or anticipate.* Your environment dictates a much slower, calmer pace.

Sitting up, you take in the view. The miles stretch before you. Twinkling sand the colour of spun gold fills your field of vision. Dunes and hollows undulate for as far as the eye can see. Their soft ripples beckon, and you rise to your feet. Your fingertips grasp for the sky and you feel the delicious pull in your spine as you stretch every muscle. Then slowly you begin to move. Behind you, rocky outcrops jut into the skyline; dusted with white sand, they glisten. You see clumps of tumbleweed in the distance; tossed by the breeze, they have no direction. They simply wait to be propelled by the elements. You imagine how wonderful that would be, to have no expectations, no frustrations, to *let nature dictate your course.*

Zig-zag patterns form in the sand as you walk. It's as if the ground beneath your feet shifts with every footfall. You'd expect the heat to overwhelm you, but instead it's a comfort, soothing away aches and pains, helping you to release the things you no longer need. Its presence is nurturing. In the distance you see more rocks, littered with cacti. Patches of emerald green, they stand out against the burnished stone. The landscape is forever changing; from Sahara sands to the desolate Mojave, it is made up of every wild and empty space in your mind. You sense there is something coming, a message just for you, but there is no need to push. *It will happen when it happens.*

Instead of heading full-pelt towards the rocks, you stand, breathe, watch as the sky in the distance begins to transform. The sun is gradually setting and each second brings a new shade. Burnt orange with rust-tipped edges gently merges to soft red and then a deep mauve pink; the desert night is a cloak of colour. A rustle from behind attracts your attention and you turn, doing a small pirouette on the spot. There, peeking between the rocks, you see him. His eyes are fixed on you. His honey-coloured fur stands out against the steel grey of the rocks and the purple sky.

'Coyote.' The word slips softly from your lips.

You know the stories, the legends of this wily creature and his exploits, but in this moment, he looks so peaceful. *There is no rush to do anything.* He watches you, and you watch him. There is a message in this silent exchange, a symbolism that only you can understand and as *your inner wisdom grows with every breath*, the meaning comes to you.

Furtive Coyote, always on the lookout for mischief, impatient for fun, and yet here he is happy to be doing nothing, to simply wait for the right moment to act. He knows he cannot force things to happen. *Everything has a time and a place.*

All he can do is *be present in this moment, and let nature take its course. What will be will be.*

'Wherever you lead, I will follow,' you say to him, 'and if you go nowhere, then I will stay. *There is no rush.*'

The words flow from you, and you mean them. Coyote nods, his silver eyes shine with understanding. Then he turns and stalks away. You follow, taking huge strides to make up the space between you. He fades into the golden sands, his shape melting into the dust, and when you reach the same spot, you feel yourself slipping away from the wilderness. Your body sifts into the brittle earth. Each grain of sand, falling into the cracks until the landscape is once more empty; a desert of dreams within your sleeping mind.

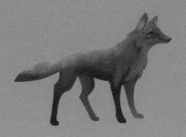

Affirmations

'There is no rush.'

'Everything happens at the right time for me.'

'Patience fills my soul.'

'My inner wisdom grows with every breath.'

Boost your mindset

Develop a deep well of patience and wisdom with this easy ritual.

If you have a garden, find a patch of soil and sit beside it. If not, you can use a plant pot filled with soil. You will also need some seeds of your choice.

Close your eyes and take a few deep breaths. Imagine a beam of light travelling down from the sky, hitting the top of your head and surging through you. Picture this light flowing into your hands and along your fingertips, infusing you with creative energy. Open your eyes and dip the fingers of both hands deep into the soil. Sift the earth rhythmically through your fingers, as if you're adding air to this earthy mixture. As you do this repeat the chant, 'I am at one with the universe and part of a much bigger picture.' Sow the seeds, then cover lightly with the soil. To finish, water them, and as you do this say 'My patience grows, like the seeds I sow.'

The physical activity of sowing and then nurturing the seeds re-enforces the idea that you also nurture qualities like patience and understanding. This, combined with a powerful affirmation that is repeated when the seeds are watered, helps to reprogram the way you think and feel.

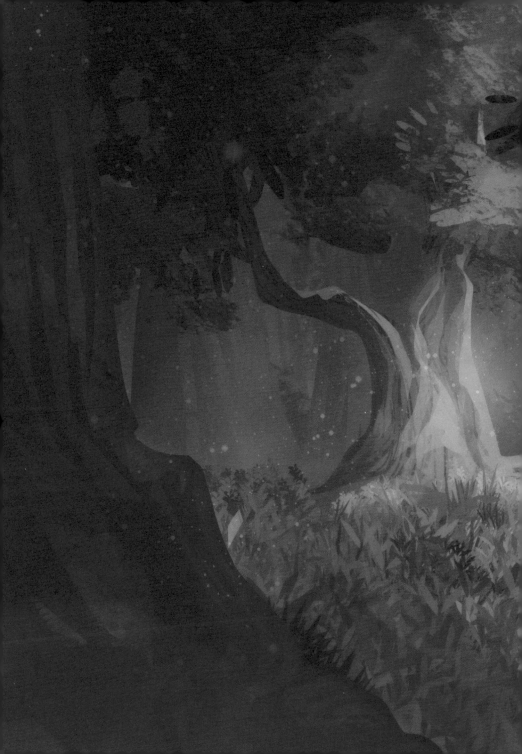

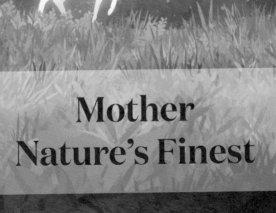

Mother
Nature's Finest

△

Boost self-esteem

—

Help you love yourself and appreciate the world around you

Imagine standing on a carpet of wildflowers, a meadow that stretches in every direction. A gentle breeze brushes your cheeks, daubing them with colour. Invisible fingers tousle your hair, and *you feel alive in every way*. You drink it all in, taking a deep breath as you survey the landscape. There's a dip to your left as the expanse of grass gives way to a cluster of trees, a thick coppice and a place of adventure. Steeped in mystery, it calls to you and you know what you must do.

You turn away from the meadow, heading down the slope to the dense woods. *Infused with energy, you stride forwards*. One foot after the other, you could almost be gliding towards your destination. It's as if the earth is carrying you. Each footfall beats in time with the rhythm of your heart. The sun, though still in the sky, is beginning to drop, casting shades of rose gold across the vista. Evening draws in and brings with it a sense of calm. You let out a sigh and soften your chest. You feel so relaxed as you near the undergrowth. Trees like sentinels stand tall at your approach, the ripples of bark upon each trunk beg to be touched and you can't resist the urge to connect with these ancient oaks. What stories must they hold within their branches? What memories must they treasure? In that brief exchange of hand and patina, you feel that wonder.

Slipping between bush and shrub you step into the heart of the wood, and feel instantly cocooned, as if you have tumbled into an enchanted realm. The canopy of trees shields you. Mother Nature has taken you under her wing. You continue to walk, drawn to the heart of this ancient forest. You feel dense vegetation beneath your feet, cushioning each step. You smell fern and leaf, moss damp with dew. Overhead birdsong heralds your arrival and in the distance something moves. It's too quick for human eyes, and you ponder the nature of this unseen companion. Are they animal, fey or both; a piece of magic come to join you on your journey? Your heart skips a beat and *excitement flows through you.*

In the distance you see a small clearing. A stream of light filters through the trees to highlight this spot, and you know it's where you need to be. Tendrils of sunlight dance before your eyes and you spin with delight, bathed in the warmth of the evening sun. You take a moment and catch your breath. The enormous oak behind you takes your weight and you lean into it. Breathing deeply, you feel the energy of the tree seeping into your spine. Spider-thin roots stretch from the soles of your feet, plunging deep into the earth. They anchor you in place, holding you safe as you contemplate the power of this place. *You feel completely calm and grounded. There is nothing else but this moment, here and now. Nurtured by nature.*

Up ahead you see movement again, and slowly your companion from earlier emerges. It's a stag with a coat the colour of the moon, shimmering antlers and eyes that seem to gaze into your soul. It moves towards you and you sense magic, rich and otherworldly. Gracefully the stag lowers its antlers allowing you to stroke its forehead. Then after a minute it moves closer and head touching brow, you are united. It looks at you as if to say 'We are one and the same, you and I. Perfect as we are.'

'Perfect as I am,' you think. The words echo in your mind as you enjoy this feeling of closeness. The stag steps back and nods, as if to affirm its point and there's a moment of silent understanding between you. Then without warning, he is gone, blown away by the wind as if he were made of blossom. It doesn't matter that you can no longer see him. You can feel him in your heart, and his message remains.

Gradually, and when you're ready, you move once more. This time in the direction of the meadow you first came from. It's getting dark and you know it's time to leave. Time to restore yourself with sleep like the rest of the land. The towering trees release you safely back into the world. They watch as you climb the hill that takes you home. With each footstep you feel more relaxed. With each breath you repeat your mantra, 'Perfect as I am.'

In the distance, illuminated by the moon, a solitary stag stands; a piece of old magic from those ancient woodlands and a time when animals and humans spoke the same language. He watches you go, one of Mother Nature's finest, then like a sprinkling of stardust he disappears into the night.

Affirmations

—

'Perfect as I am.'

'I am nurtured by nature.'

'Magic lives in my soul.'

'I give love, I receive love, I am love.'

Boost your mindset

Try this, anytime, anywhere, when you need an instant confidence boost!

As you stand, lengthen your spine and relax your shoulders. Feel the weight drop into your feet and imagine you're supported by an enormous oak tree. Its trunk keeps you upright and gives you strength and confidence. You lean against the bark and feel the warm energy seeping beneath your skin. Your feet are anchored to the floor, by roots that grow from each sole and spread deep beneath the earth. You are connected to nature and ready for anything!

Good posture generates positive energy. It affects the way we think and feel and allows us to breathe correctly, which in turn floods the system with oxygen, providing focus and clarity.

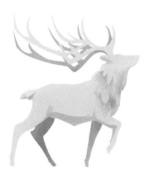

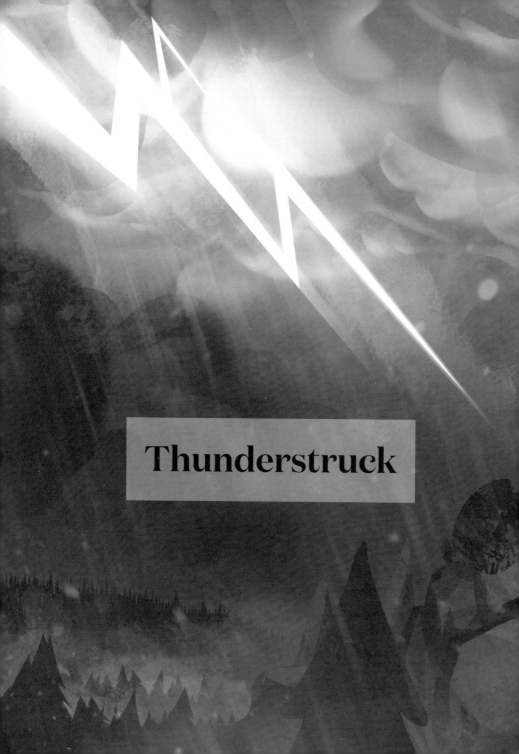

Thunderstruck

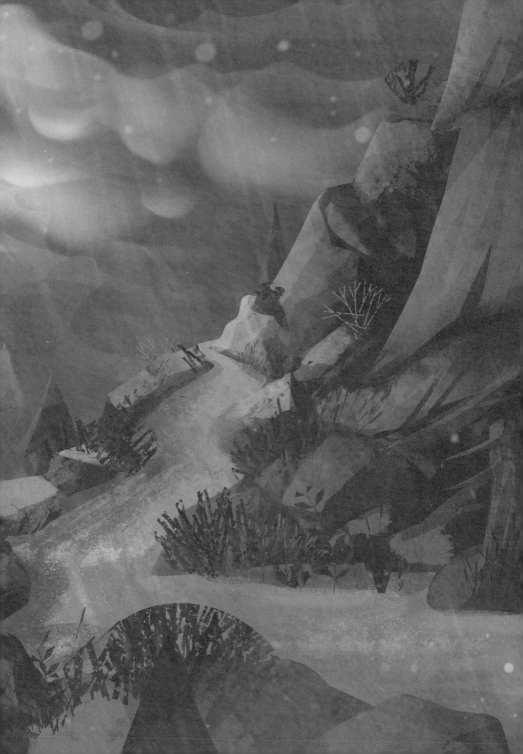

A GUIDED NARRATIVE TO:

Build inner reserves of strength

———

Promote determination

The crowds are heaving, clustered together at the starting line. Each runner is focused on the task in hand, bristling with energy and ready to take on the mountain challenge. They have years of training behind them and are prepared for every eventuality. You stand there too, shoulder to shoulder with the gathered athletes, proudly displaying your number upon your chest. You know what you must do, what you must achieve.

The mountain rises before you; a dark, foreboding mass, it seems insurmountable, but *nothing is impossible*. You may not be the best or the fittest, but your drive is enough to carry you forwards. You have a secret, something nobody else knows. It's a superpower that you can unleash when the time is right.

The starting gun sounds and you're off, gaze fixed on the pinnacle. In your mind you have already reached the top. You've seen it many times in your head. The sheer exaltation as you breathe the mountain air, as the wind buffets you. Shivers snake down your spine and your entire body is pumped.

You can do this!

You shake your fist in the air, as if in triumph.

'*Whatever I set my mind to, I achieve!*'

The crowd roars with applause. Everyone knows you're a winner.

Steadily the path inclines, working each muscle to its max. Your legs feel heavy and your breath short, but this is only the beginning. There are miles to go and you must push through the pain. You are no longer aware of anyone else in the race. It feels like you are on your own on this mountain; a solitary stranger battling the elements. Fear taints your thoughts and you wonder what will happen if you don't make it to the top, if you fall, or worse still give up, but you know better.

'*I will have my victory,*' you whisper.

The ground dips and twists, getting steeper with every beat of your heart. The billowing wind shakes you, making each footfall a precarious dance but still you continue.

'I *will* have my victory.'

Willpower is crucial to your success. The sky darkens, huge angry rain clouds cluster giving you their worst, the showers come down and in seconds you are soaked to the bone. A single dart of lightning blasts through the shadows, then another. You feel like this attack is aimed at you and there is no escape. You are trapped, exposed upon the mountainside, an easy target. But then you realize the lightning is not your enemy. It's a force of nature, just like you.

Suddenly you're infused with vitality, as if you've been supercharged with electricity. You feel the switch flick inside, as tiny shoots of light spread through your entire being. In your mind you don a superhero costume. You see it materializing, forming a second golden skin to cover your own. Your legs feel loose, free to bend and stretch, to push on in huge leaps and bounds. Your chest expands and fuelled by the extra oxygen you move faster and faster. Your arms part the air, making you even more dynamic and soon you're motoring up the mountain, leaving everyone behind. Soaring, barely touching the ground as you go.

Superhuman, supernatural, faster than the lightning above your head. You can see the ground rushing past you. Rocks crumble as you skim above them. You're a shark in the ocean, sleek and focused on your aim. Ahead you see the tip of the mountain, it's within your grasp and in moments you're there. It's as if thinking about doing it is enough. *The power of your mind is enough.*

You've made it!

You knew you would, and it's just as you imagined. The view is spectacular, and you feel on top of the world. Mist crowds you, clambering close because you are the champion. There's a rock protruding from the mount, like a stone throne it's the perfect fit and you sit and enjoy the moment. Below the ground is a patchwork of colour, and you realize how far you have come. This is proof that you can achieve anything you set your mind to. A blaze of sun parts the clouds, showering you in warmth. Nature says well done; you deserve this.

The arduous climb is not forgotten, but you realize it's part of the prize, the most important bit. *The journey is where you learned how to fly.* You built your resolve and fought with tenacity to reach the summit. The race was tough, but its gift is endurance.

You have inner reserves of strength at your fingertips.

With this thought fixed in your mind, you begin your descent, the slope giving you the momentum you need to glide back to earth and face your next challenge.

Affirmations

'I am victorious in all things.'

'The power of my mind is enough.'

'I always reach my destination.'

'Endurance is my super-power.'

Boost your mindset

Think of a time when you achieved something that you're proud of. This could be passing an exam, getting a new job or promotion, or even something practical like decorating your home.

Imagine you are watching a film of the experience in your mind and when you reach the moment of victory, freeze the frame and press your index finger and thumb together in a pinching motion.

Say out loud or in your head 'I can do anything I set my mind to.' Repeat this process every day for a week to re-enforce the action and thought pattern. Whenever you need extra reserves of strength and determination, pinch your index finger and thumb together, and you'll be instantly reminded of your awesomeness!

Drawing on a powerful memory and combining it with a simple action reprograms the mind. You'll be able to recreate the feelings associated with the experience anytime, simply by performing the physical action.

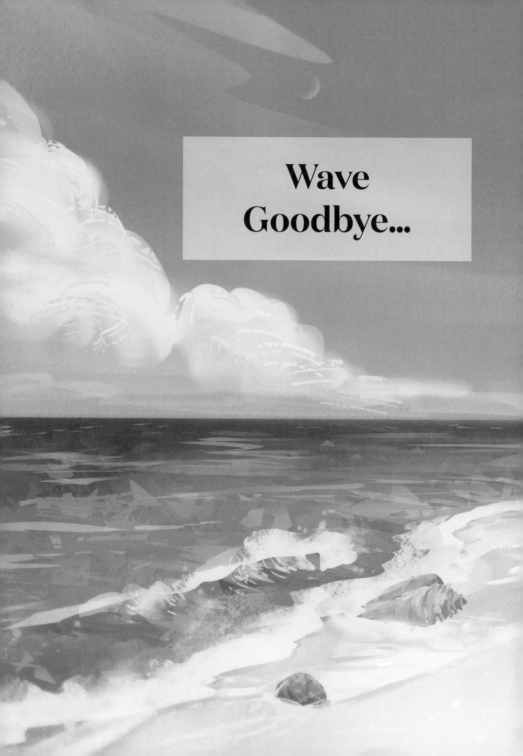

Wave Goodbye...

A GUIDED NARRATIVE TO:

Promote self-healing

—

Help you release the past

The sun kisses your forehead as you lay upon the sand, it bathes you in adoration. This beach is what you deserve; a break from the everyday and some time to relax and reflect. Comforting rays brush against your skin while a gentle breeze ruffles your hair. You are alone, but not lonely. You hear the sounds of children playing, splashing in the sea. People in the distance talking and laughing, but they are getting further and further away with every breath, until they're just fragments, echoes drifting along the shoreline. The silence gives you perspective and your mind feels suddenly alert and ready for its next quest. *Life is sweet and you are in a good place, a safe space.* This is your version of paradise.

In and out you breathe, in time with the ebb and flow of the ocean. On and on, in a continual loop, a cycle of rise and fall as you unwind. You can feel the stress falling from your shoulders, dissolving into the golden sand. Slowly you rise, until you're standing tall. Stretching up on your tip-toes, you imagine grasping the sun with both hands, pulling this fiery orb into your chest. You smile.

All is good in your world right now.

Before you is the sea; a swell of vibrant sapphire with threads of emerald and the lightest aquamarine at the surface. A beautiful boundless beast, it moves in giant rolls and you wonder what it would be like to go with that flow. *To surrender to the waves.*

You walk forwards, your focus on the horizon. Deep azure blue washes over you. The shrill call of a sea bird captures your attention if only for a moment, then you are back, gaze fixed on the middle of the ocean, on the secrets beneath the watery brine. Your feet sink into the sand, swallowed by the glorious gold dust of those that went before you. The earth becomes moist, a clay-like substance that moulds to the shape of each foot. Still you move forward fixed on your goal, on the cool trickle at the edge of the shore. You want to feel water lapping at your toes, hungrily seeking out each one in a bid to claim it. Soon you are there, paddling by the edge. Able to feel the refreshing nip of the water as you stroll along the beach.

The sun takes your breath away and you shield your eyes, as all the colours of the vista take on new life. Golds that veer towards amber catch your eye; palms the darkest green, they make you think of saturated rainforests, and the soft baby blue of the sky, an artist's palette painted to perfection. You sigh and let out any remaining stress. All worry is banished in this place. *Calm is the only thing you feel.*

You breathe in this moment. Finally, you understand that this is all you have. The present is a gift. You are ready to let go of the past. To release the pain you've been holding onto. You stop in your tracks. Turn to face the sea. Ever welcoming, it rushes towards you in the crest of a wave. You step back, making a mark with your toe. Then into the pliable sand you work, crafting a symbol to represent all of the hurt, guilt and fear that you feel. All of the things that have been holding you back. You make your mark upon the earth and pour all of those emotions into it. Then, when you are ready, you look towards the horizon once more.

'I give this to you,' you say.

'I release my pain. I let it all go.'

The ocean smiles. Runs to greet you again. The waves eager to wash away the hurt and transform it into light. Smoothly and swiftly the sea heals, wiping the slate clean and stealing the symbol that you have made from the sand. In that one motion the pain is gone, swept away and you are left lighter, more radiant than you have ever been before.

Your heart leaps, and suddenly you feel a pull to go deeper, to submerge in the watery depths and feel that healing energy surround you. Taking long strides, the waves part at your touch. The sea accepts you unconditionally. Within seconds you're up to the chest, arms sweeping, propelling you forwards. Your legs are floating behind you. There is little effort involved. The ocean carries and supports every movement you make.

Light as a feather, as a thought, as a breath.

You feel totally at peace. Healed from the inside out.

Affirmations

———

'All is good, all is calm.'

'I surrender to the ebb and flow.'

'I release pain, I let it go.'

'Healing energy washes over me.'

Boost your mindset

Use the power of water to boost healing, by incorporating these top tips into your schedule.

Infuse body and soul with healing energy throughout the day by sipping water. This will keep you hydrated and also help you to remain focused in challenging situations. Imagine that each mouthful is imbued with positive energy, which surges through your body as you drink.

If you need an extra boost of vitality, run the cold tap and place your wrists underneath the flow of water for at least a minute. As you do this picture a stream of white light travelling up each arm and around your entire body. Breathe deeply and relax.

Alternatively fill the sink with cold water and submerge your hands. Close your eyes and imagine you are dipping your hands into the sea.

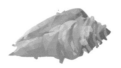

Running cold water on your wrists lowers the body's core temperature and heart rate and helps to reduce levels of cortisol, the stress hormone. This coupled with a relaxing visualization will make you feel instantly calmer.

Wave Goodbye...

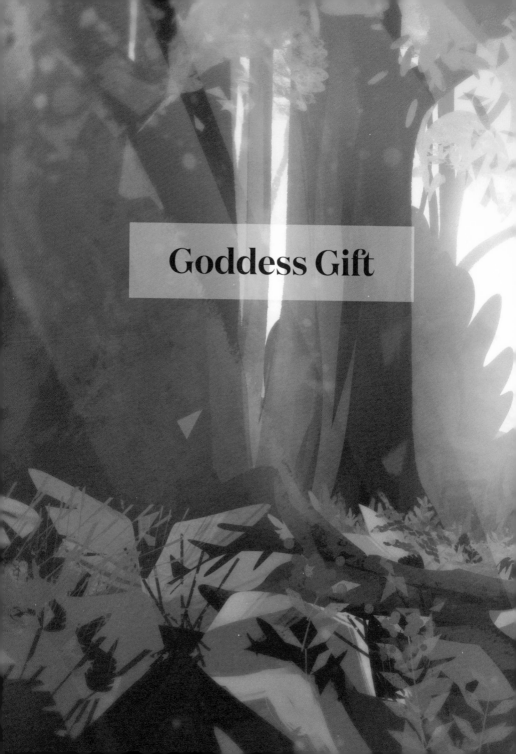

Goddess Gift

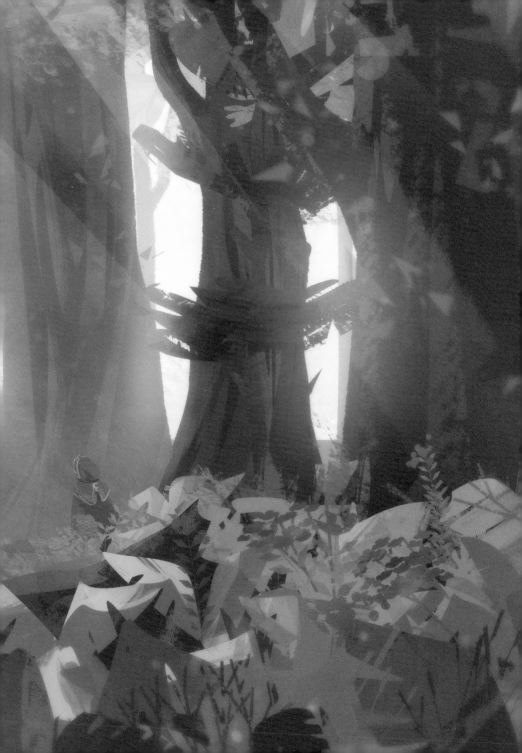

△

Connect to your higher self

—

Improve intuitive skills

You are standing barefoot in the centre of a woody copse. Warm light streams through the trees, casting auburn rays in every direction. Moss cushions your feet, and you feel light as a feather, as if you could float up to the tips of the trees and dance in the forest canopy. It's autumn, and the mellow scent of honey and damp soil hangs in the air. It wraps you in a shawl of crisp and colourful leaves. As you take in your surroundings, you notice that they are already changing. Clusters of berries darken before your eyes. The late fruits of summer are ripening upon the vine. Ferns unfurl and then snake delicately around the trunks of trees. Wherever you turn your attention your energy goes with it, bringing transformation.

Your heart flutters and you place both hands over your chest. *The gossamer wings of your intuition take flight, and you feel a pull deep within*, a need to move further into this mystical realm. You take a step and the leaves crunch beneath your bare feet. The rustling sound as you move fills you with anticipation, and then you see it. An orb, the colour of the brightest ruby, spins before your eyes then slips between the slender pines. Excited, you follow, skipping in a zig-zag pattern as the light twists and turns. Soon you are running, leaping over twisted roots and pinecones, the autumn breeze nipping at your heels. You can feel thousands of eyes upon you. The creatures of the forest watch and delight in your journey. And there are other eyes too, twinkling and fey; nature spirits that track your every move with interest. You can sense their presence, and as you move, you hear them whisper words of encouragement.

The land dips beneath your feet, and soon you find yourself in a clearing. It's a small glade surrounded by ancient oaks, and there in the centre is a woman wearing a cloak of fire. As you get closer you see that what you thought were flames is really a patchwork of burnt orange leaves, moulded to her skin. Her moon-shaped face beams at your approach and she opens her arms to welcome you.

'I have been waiting,' she says.

You walk towards her and notice the roots curling in her hair; they form tendrils that fall about her shoulders. Her cloak is made of dried leaves and acorns, strings of burnished conkers trail at its hem. She holds out a hand, extending her arm like a stem reaching towards the sunlight.

'I have a gift for you,' she smiles.

You reach towards her, your hand slipping into hers and in that moment a white rose bursts from your palm. You watch in awe as the flower opens, each petal sending sparks of light into the air. Tendrils of fern wrap around your arm, spreading up to stretch gently around your shoulders and down the other side. A cloak of golden feathers gathers about you and a crown of ivy sits upon your head.

You are connected to the earth. You feel every movement, every breath that is taken. You can hear each word, each sound from a crow's wings in flight, to the soft beating of your heart. You instinctively know your calling, who you are and what you must do, what your gift is and how you can use it to help others. *Your thoughts connect you to your higher self*, the seat of your intuition. The veil that separates worlds has lifted and you can see and feel that which was once invisible.

Your psychic senses are primed.

The shadows that slid between the trees now shimmer into view, they are sylph-like beings formed of air, spirits of the wood. The wizened trunks of the trees ripple with energy. They emanate a soft glow, an aura of light that encases the timber, and the leaves too. The plants and the creatures that crawl and fly, they all have an aura that you can see. You don't need to understand what is happening, you know within that *you have the power to feel and read the signs and symbols.*

Your intuition is your guide in all things.

You turn to thank your companion, the beautiful being that has given you this gift, but she is gone. And then you realize that she is a part of you: the higher self, where divine wisdom is found. Always present, always willing to assist, you can tap into this well of knowledge whenever you need to. You place your hands palms-down over your heart and breathe, in and out, in and out...

... in time with the earth, in sync with the divine, and at one with your intuition.

Affirmations

———

'All the answers I need are within me.'

'My intuition is my guide.'

'I am at one with the earth and the divine.'

'My higher self leads the way.'

Boost your mindset

Your intuition speaks to you through signs, symbols, and feelings. Learn to recognize this language and understand the deeper meaning with this exercise.

Close your eyes and place both hands over your heart. Breathe deeply for a couple of minutes to calm and clear the mind.

Notice how you feel – do you have any strange sensations in your chest, or stomach? Does an image or a feeling spring to mind? Allow thoughts to come and go and continue to breathe deeply. When you've finished, make a note in a special journal of anything you remember.

Practise this for five minutes every day and continue to write up your thoughts and feelings. After a while you'll notice a pattern emerging, you'll see that certain sensations have more meaning and that words or symbols are connected. You'll recognize a feeling when it happens, for example the tingle of excitement in your stomach when something good is about to occur. Over time you'll be able to decipher the language of your intuition and you'll instinctively know what each message means.

When you pay attention to your intuition, through the medium of your thoughts and feelings, you become more in tune with the higher self, and your spiritual life path.

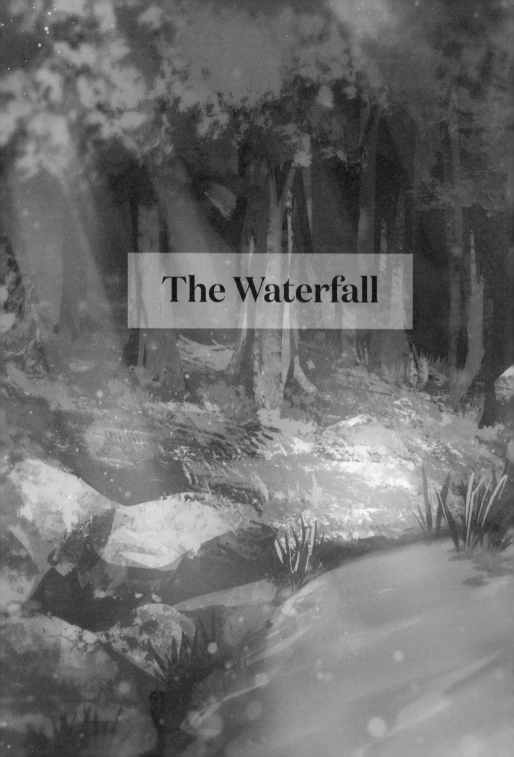

The Waterfall

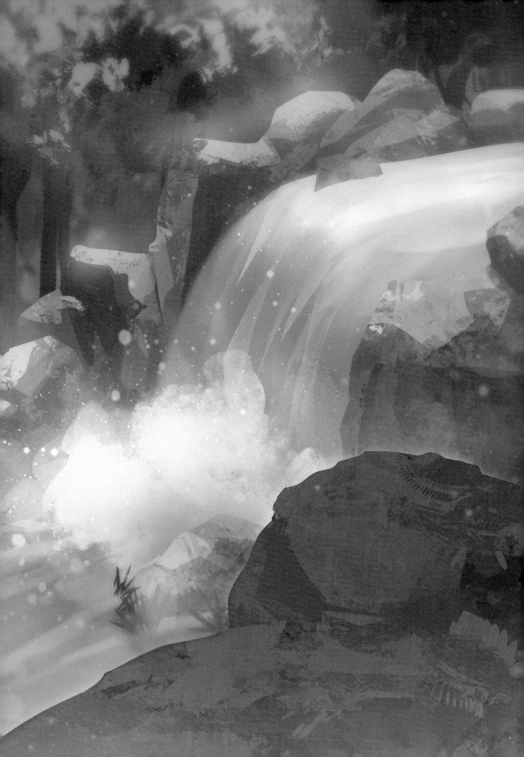

A GUIDED NARRATIVE TO:

Restore vitality

—

Imbue passion and energy

Before you, the water flows. You drink in the sight and sound of it rushing, beating a path from the brow of the hill down to the forest floor. It cascades over the edge, tumbling down to create the most beautiful waterfall you have ever seen. It takes your breath away. You watch as it pools, a frothy white mass that loops and swirls down the mountainside. As you stand halfway up, you listen to the sounds, the whoosh and the whirr, the magical trickles that dance like musical notes above your head, and you long to be a part of the symphony. The water looks so pure and inviting. Like liquid crystal, it glistens in the afternoon sun. Everything it touches becomes more vibrant, as if lit from the inside.

You climb a little higher, feeling your way along each piece of rock until you are standing directly beneath this spectacle. A spray of fine droplets peppers your skin. Tiny pinpricks of moisture that make each pore tingle with joy.

You're infused with energy.

Your body feels almost fluid, as if you could change shape and navigate any landscape. Your mind too is alive and active. New ideas flood your vision, and *you feel suddenly awake and ready to take on the world.*

The waterfall continues to rush past, charged with a mission to reach the swell of the stream below. Nothing stands in its way. Nothing can stop it; such is the power and the potential of nature. You long to feel the same, to be charged with vigour. You reach out your hands, let the water hit your skin. It pelts each palm, wrapping around your fingers then slipping through them before you can grasp it. It taunts you, begs you to follow, to join in with this watery dance and let gravity take hold.

There is no decision to be made, no thought or preparation.

You are a dynamic soul and, in this moment, you can do anything.

Stretching your arms to a point above your head, you dip forwards and plunge, joining forces with the waterfall. You are a darting, diving shadow amongst the sparkling stream. Svelte and lithe, you twist and turn, letting the water animate you. It's an easy passage and with each sweep of your arms, you feel more energized and able to let go. Full of verve and passion, you glide, not knowing or caring the direction, just *delighting in your own vitality*.

A surge of adrenalin powers through you, and you skim the surface during your downward descent. Your body ripples, pouring forwards until you become part of a much bigger body of water. Increasing in mass and drive, you are almost there, almost ready to hit the ground running. You take a gulp of air, drinking it down deep. *The energy is exhilarating!*

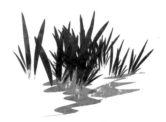

And then it happens, instant and invigorating; you reach the bottom, plunging beneath the glistening surface. You made it! You swam the waterfall, plummeted its dazzling depths and let it seep into your heart. The momentum of the fall has left you elated. For a moment you tread water and catch your breath. The cool stream gathers around you and you feel refreshed. Your spine bristles and your mind fizzes with energy. If you were despondent before, now you are renewed. The switch has been flicked and *you are bubbling with anticipation.*

You gaze up at the waterfall and find that you can no longer see where it starts or ends, how high it is or how it was created. It's as if the gushing rivulets are a cosmic gift from the universe. As if the heavens have opened and allowed the elixir of life to fall to earth. You realize then how blessed you are. Every day offers the chance of renewal, the opportunity for rebirth and to feel this invigoration. All you have to do is invite positive energy into your life.

Be open, be brave, and embrace your vibrance.

Slowly, you rise from the water, pulling yourself onto the damp mossy bank. You shake the droplets from your hair and marvel at your glistening skin. Upon your face is a wide smile. Your heart beats with passion, and you glow from head to toe.

Vitality is restored.

Affirmations

———

'I am infused with energy.'

'I am a dynamic soul and I shine with vitality.'

'Every day I am renewed.'

'Vibrance oozes from every pore.'

Boost your mindset

Boost your vitality by connecting to the invigorating energy of the waterfall. Practise this visualization anytime and anywhere, whenever you need a pick-me-up.

Take a moment to relax, breathe deeply and calm your mind. Close your eyes and imagine you're standing beneath a glorious waterfall, like the one in the story. You can feel the shimmering water flowing over you, hitting the top of your head and cascading over your shoulders. The tiny droplets are infused with magical energy, and they shine like diamonds. As you breathe in, imagine the vibrant water passing through the top of your head, flooding your entire body with vitality. As you breathe out, picture the water flowing freely from the soles of your feet into a stream. Stretch each breath out for as long as possible and continue this loop of inhaling the diamond-bright energy and releasing it back to nature.

Do this for five minutes every morning to feel energized and ready for anything!

In folklore, the waterfall is a symbol of rejuvenation. It's associated with spiritual cleansing and connected to the crown chakra, located at the top of the head. The combination of the symbol and the breathing technique helps to cleanse and renew mind, body and spirit.

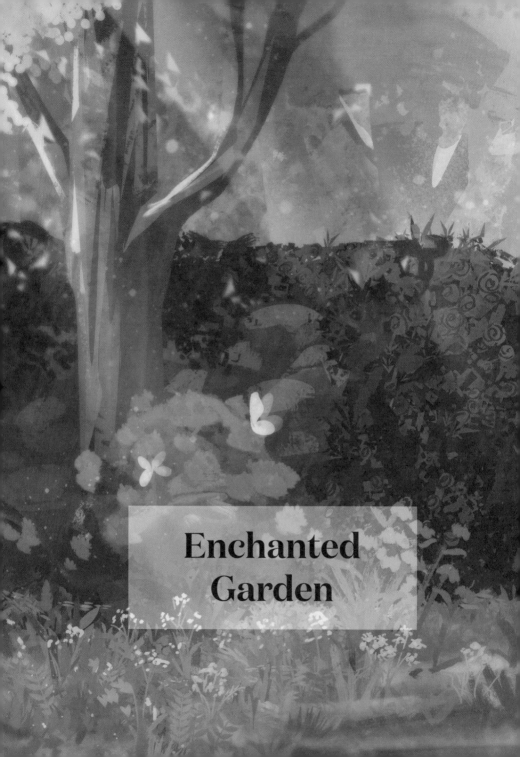

Enchanted
Garden

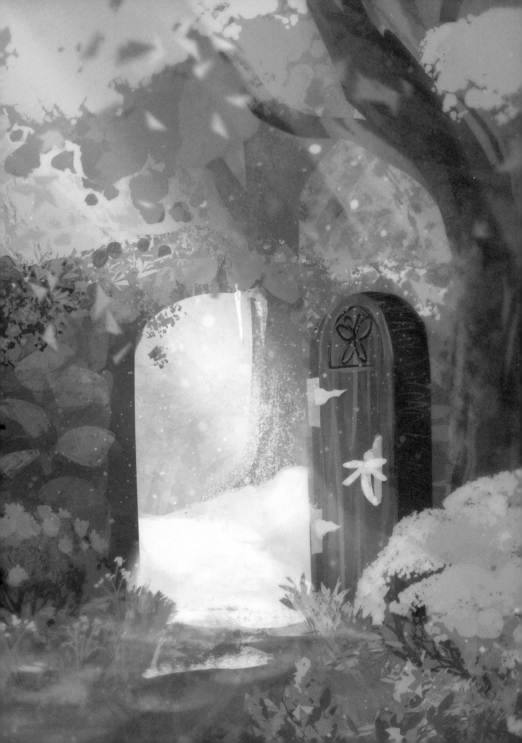

A GUIDED NARRATIVE TO:

Restore balance

———

Help you embrace the
ebb and flow of life

It's a beautiful summer's evening. The scent of honeysuckle fills the air. You are walking by the side of a walled garden. Climbing tea roses scale the stone; they sprawl in every direction, peppering the wall with hints of pink, yellow and luminous white. The birds accompany you on your journey. They twitter their delicate song above your head. The path you've chosen meanders in no particular direction, but that's OK. *You feel relaxed and trust that nature will lead you where you need to be.*

Up ahead you see a door nestled in the wall. It is carved from oak and engraved with vines and butterflies. You wonder what lies behind this door, what is waiting for you on the other side. You reach out, touch the grain of the wood. It feels smooth, ancient, filled with secrets. Gently you push. The huge brass hinges of the door creak, as it glides open and you are bathed in golden sunshine.

You step forward into the light, unable at first to see anything, but gradually your sight adjusts and you take in your surroundings. You are standing in the centre of a magical garden. Fluted blooms cluster between majestic sunflowers, their vibrant faces turned upwards. Bushes littered with pretty pink and purple flowers seem to vibrate with the heavy hum of bees at work. Trees enclose the entire space, some small, just finding their first leaves, while others tower over the scene, their wide, glossy leaves cloaking the garden in a wash of deep green. Ferns trail around worn stone planters filled with pansies and petunias, while willowy irises sway in the borders. Wherever you look you see something new and delightful. The joys of summer fill your heart and you long to stay in this place forever.

But just as this thought arises, so the scenery shifts, and you find you are part of a different picture. The light flickers from summer brightness to a deeper, richer tone. There's warmth in these amber hues but also a nip to the air, a chill that seeps under your skin. The ground beneath your feet seems to ripple and then harden, and for a moment you feel out of place, unsure and unsteady. You take a breath, *draw down the energy of the earth and feel it anchoring you in place*. Just as the shrubs and trees are tethered by nature, so are you; connected to all things and in harmony with the seasons.

The leaves crisp before your eyes, the luscious emerald tones turn yellow and then lighten, becoming orange and red. Glowing fronds of autumn brightness greet you at every turn. The flowers are now almost gone, but the colour is still spectacular. Tendrils of wind ruffle your hair, picking up leaves and twigs in a swirl which dances before your eyes, but you do not move. You are rooted to the spot. *In perfect balance with the world around you.*

Then just as quickly as it first began, this symphony is over. The blaze of colour fades, and the shadows of winter sneak in. You can feel them working their way into the space before your eyes. Dark, spectral, but exquisite in the way they change the atmosphere. The leaves have disappeared. The skeletal trees strike a pose against an almost white backdrop. Plants withdraw into themselves and the soil to be replenished. All is calm, just like your breathing. A thin layer of frost adds the finishing touch, making everything glisten and the chill sets in. It gnaws at your bones and reminds you that you are alive, that you can feel and think and be energized by the icy cold, just as the warmth of the sun lifts your spirits. There is a time and a place for everything.

Light and dark, black and white. Nature is in balance.

Spring is around the corner; in a heartbeat it beckons. Beneath your feet you feel it coming. New life stirs in the womb of the earth. It trembles, and you feel a rush of excitement and anticipation at what is to come. The first shoots appear, pushing through the soil. Blades of grass spring up at every turn and you marvel at the changes. At the ebb and flow of life. Bushes unfurl, their stems filled with buds. Trees brighten, reaching for the sun as their canopy of leaves sprout and thicken.

The cycle moves on, from old to new, from yin to yang.

It is time now for you to go, but you do not leave the enchanted garden with nothing. You carry with you a thought, a truth that you will keep with you, always.

Nature is balance and you are nature.

Affirmations

———

'The earth anchors me.'

'I am in perfect balance with nature.'

'I am exactly where I need to be.'

'My mind, body and soul are in harmony.'

Boost your mindset

Restore balance and stability with this simple exercise.

Stand with your feet hip-width apart, shoulders relaxed, and chin tilted slightly upwards. Picture a thread that travels through the top of your head and down your spine. Imagine that this thread is being tugged gently and feel your spine gradually lengthening.

Turn your attention to the soles of your feet and feel the weight of your body as it's balanced equally through each leg. Bounce lightly, bending at the knees and notice how you are supported by the earth.

Draw your hands, palms together, and pull them in to your heart. Close your eyes and picture a yin yang symbol in the centre of your chest. Focus on this image for a few minutes, and breathe deeply.

The yin yang symbol is universally associated with balance; this combined with a physical exercise that focuses on posture and movement helps to promote a sense of stability and equilibrium.

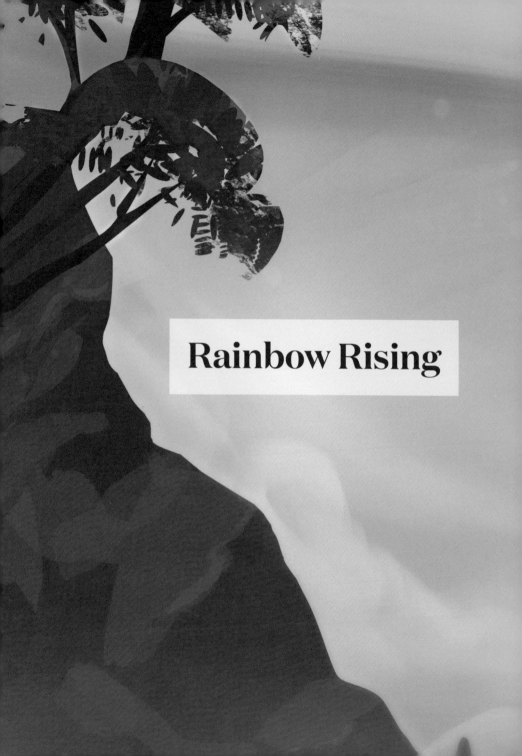

Rainbow Rising

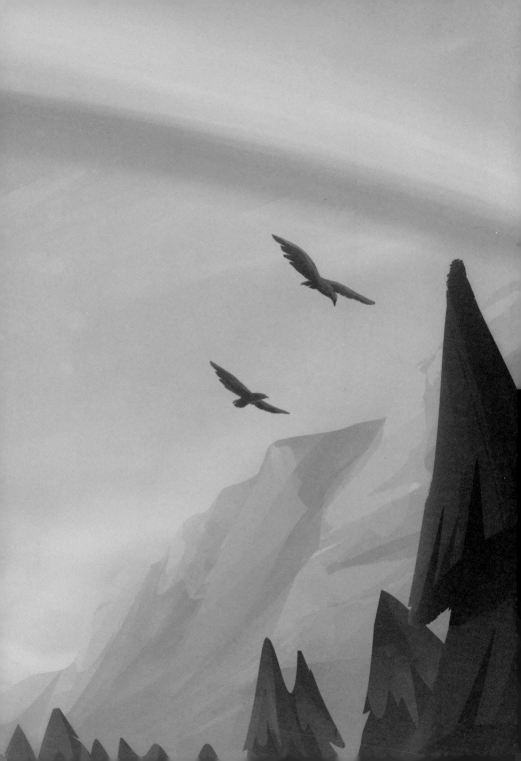

A GUIDED NARRATIVE TO:

De-stress

—

Feel relaxed and positive

You are standing in a deep valley between a cluster of giant hills, mounds of earth that penetrate the grey sky. You have been walking, the stark silence of nature your only companion. The sky is a darkening smudge above your head. The grass beneath your feet is wet and it feels as if you're standing in thick clay. You twist around, in an attempt to take in the view from all sides. Emptiness greets you. There are slopes that rise and fall in every direction, just as your breath rises and falls. You are at one with the landscape, as much a part of it as the cluster of crows sweeping above your head.

The black plume of corvids softly caws, and it feels like they're speaking directly to you, trying to attract your attention in some way. The sound gets louder, more frantic and you reach up towards them, watch as they flounce higher into the air, heading for the hill's peak. The charcoal grey of the sky is a gaping hole, offering space and tranquillity and you drink in the sight of it. It has been raining, but the sun is out now, bursting through the clouds and chasing away the last of the gloom. You smile.

Even the darkest skies can't keep the sun at bay.

Looking up, you notice intricate carvings, indents into the side of the bank and slithers of stone that jut from the earth. Birds gather upon these makeshift ledges. Flitting from one to the other in an aerial dance. They peer down at you and suddenly you long to be up there with them, to experience their realm. Above this pinnacle a rainbow forms, it's an explosion of colour and made even brighter by the fact there are two of them. You clap your hands together and make a wish at this heavenly sight.

For a moment, it feels like the world is frozen. Time stands still and there is only you and the rainbow cascading down at your feet. Glittering hues swirl around you, like a glorious tornado and you feel yourself being lifted into the air. Carried by ribbons of light, you relax into the spectrum of colour.

Your arms and shoulders feel free from tension.

The muscles in your legs melt away to nothing, and your spine extends and softens.

You breathe deeply.

Your eyelids lower and you relax your neck and throat.

The ligaments in your body feel more fluid, as you continue to float upwards.

It's as if you've become at one with the sky that surrounds you. You are a spiritual being made up of particles of light, *happy to be carried wherever the rainbow takes you.*

You close your eyes completely now and enjoy feeling as if you're made of air. A smile curves your lips. *There is no room for stress here.* No room for anything except joy. You drop your weight into your lower legs and find that you are perfectly balanced. The wind supports you, holding you upright as you float. As you open your eyes once more you see that you are surfing the rainbow, gliding gracefully along its colourful edges. Bathed in the light from each hue, you feel the colours seeping into your aura. With every long, slow breath in you drink down each shade, taking it deep into your soul. You sigh.

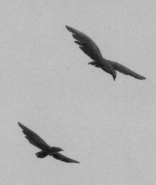

Relaxation sweeps over you as the colours resonate within.

All thoughts of the day ahead have gone. *There is no pressure to do anything.* You can simply be. The colours drape around you. They cocoon you in their brightness. The rainbow is never-ending; a bridge in the sky to a new way of being, a new, more relaxed you. The landscape moves beneath you, and although you are still a part of it, *you feel removed, able to carry a sense of calm through your day.*

The distance between the earth and the sky is like the distance you now feel from the things which cause you tension. Stretching your arms out at your sides, you let the breeze buffet you, and imagine for a second that you have wings that can lift you up, anytime, anywhere. The rainbow dips, and you begin to slide back down to earth. It is a gradual motion, and you land delicately, as if you've never moved from the spot.

The smile is still upon your face and as you continue on your walk, you feel the rainbow, it entwines around you, bathing you in tranquillity. No matter where you are or what happens during your day, *you will always hold serenity in your soul.*

Affirmations

———

'I hold serenity in my soul.'

'I am cocooned in a rainbow of light.'

'Calmness covers me.'

'I soar above the stress.'

Boost your mindset

When you're feeling under stress and need to calm down and distance yourself from a situation, try this on-the-spot visualization.

To begin, find an image of a rainbow and focus on it for a couple of minutes. When you're ready, close your eyes and imagine you're sitting beneath the arch of the rainbow in your picture. You can feel the warmth of the sun on the top of your head, infusing you with peace.

With every breath in and out, the rainbow extends, its colours spreading and becoming more vibrant. Continue to breathe deeply, and picture the rainbow gradually descending from the sky, until it's touching your head. Slowly it wraps around you, covering you from head to toe in an array of vivid hues. You are drenched in all the colours of the rainbow. When you inhale, you take in the uplifting energy of each ray. As you exhale you release all the fear, worry and stress back into the air.

When you are ready, emerge from the rainbow, give your limbs a shake and do a mental check of your body. You should feel light, centred and relaxed.

Slow, deep breathing calms the body and the mind, and is particularly powerful when coupled with a visualization using colour and light.

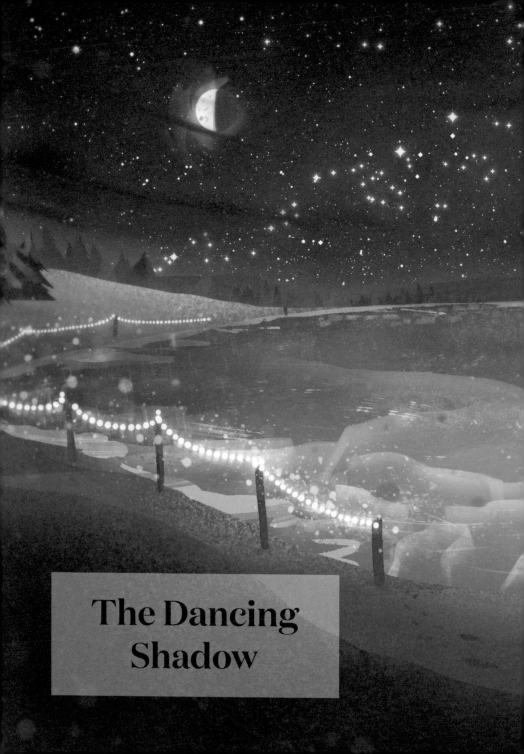

The Dancing Shadow

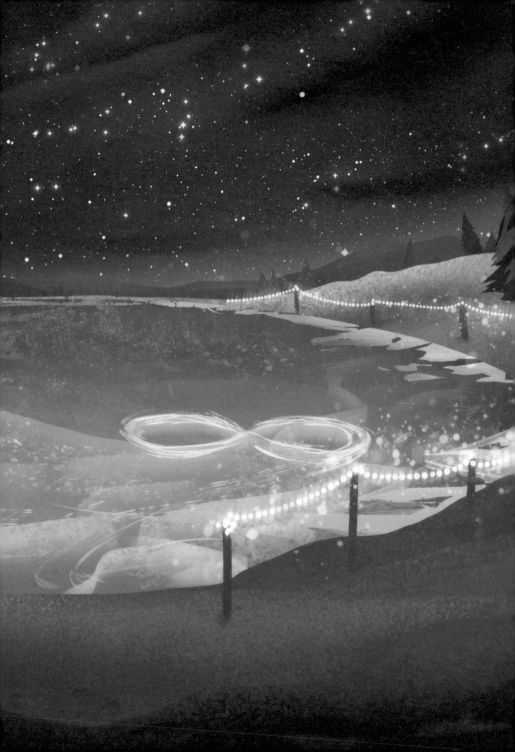

A GUIDED NARRATIVE TO:

Open your heart

———

Encourage forgiveness

Glaciers of ice cut like diamonds command this winter landscape. Everything is covered in a thick layer of snow; it glistens like icing sugar underneath the stars. Lanterns twinkle in the distance and you can see fairy lights strung above your head, surrounding a giant lake of ice. The skaters have long since left, but the lights still shimmer red, gold, blue and green. This translucent ballroom begs to be used, to feel the delicate patter of feet spinning and turning upon its surface. The hazy glow of the sunset is your backdrop, night is merging with day and the colours blend in marble swirls of burnt orange and purple. The scene before you melts your heart. You long to be the solitary dancer, to take flight upon the floor. The universe hears your plea and propels you forwards.

Looking down at your feet you find you have skates on. Snug and supportive, it feels like you've been wearing them all your life. And while you might never have taken to the ice before, it comes naturally, as if you were born to it. Surging forward you glide with grace, creating a sweeping circle with your blades. Your body sways, taking each movement in your stride. You loop and then loop again, making a continuous figure of eight, the symbol of infinity. Just as life goes on and on, so does this dance upon the ice. Weaving and dipping, you extend your leg out behind you, your arms stretching up to the darkening sky. *Everything is in perfect harmony.* Every part of you is working to create this balance.

Each step that you take builds a pattern in the ice, a roadmap to follow. As you push through with each skate, you push all of those harmful emotions you've been harbouring away. You smooth the path before you, making it easy to navigate. With every manoeuvre you become more open, not only to the dance but to life itself. Your heart softens and you feel warm inside. There is no need for harsh protective walls, for thorns or thickets to keep intruders at bay. It's time to allow yourself to feel, to breathe through your emotions and express them in the way you perform.

You leap in the air, half expecting to crash because you've never done anything like this before. Instead you land with poise, a bright smile upon your face. Love flows through you; love for yourself and love for others, love for your nearest and dearest and for those you've never met. It is then that you notice you are not alone upon the ice. A shadowy figure has joined you in the dance. It's a shape you recognize well.

Holding out both hands, your mystery partner seeks forgiveness and while they will not show their face, you know who it is, who is seeking your absolution. Linking arms, you lead them to the infinity symbol and together you loop the loop, in unison. Every movement is in time, as if you were fashioned as a pair. Above you the stars turn up their brightness and the moon casts a loving glow. Gone are the rosy hues of earlier, replaced by shades of blue, from ocean deep to charcoal black. *You feel protected, ready to open your heart and let go.*

One final tracing of the figure of eight and you're face to face with the masked skater. Eye to eye, except their facial features remain obscured.

'I forgive you,' you say, cupping your heart as you speak.

Silence cuts the ice between you, and again you whisper, *'I let the pain go and open my heart to you.'*

The stranger remains motionless, sheathed in darkness. You move closer. Hands seeking the truth, you lift the mask to reveal the hidden dancer. You always knew who it was, so it's no surprise to see the mirror image of yourself staring back.

'I forgive myself,' the dancer replies and in that instant you feel weightless.

Lights dance before your eyes, thousands of tiny flickering sparks that come from nowhere and cloud your vision. You shield your eyes and then as the scene before you fades, you see that everything has changed. The darting lights have gone, your shadow self has vanished into the night.

One last time you circle the rink, only now you seem to float, each skate hovering in mid-air. You are a feather upon the wind, free at last to go with the flow. You forgive yourself as you forgive others, and in doing so, you break the chains and create a new story – one with you at the centre of it.

This is the beginning of your fairy tale.

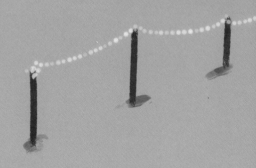

Affirmations

———

'I forgive myself.'

'My heart is open to give and receive love.'

'Everything is in harmony, in my life.'

'Forgiveness sets me free.'

Boost your mindset

If you're angry with someone and need to forgive them, use this simple exercise to release the pain and move on.

To start, write a letter to this person. Pour all your emotions into it and tell them how you feel. Then light a white candle and as it burns, pass the paper through the flame. Collect the ash in a bowl, and scatter outside.

Next, close your eyes and picture yourself standing face to face with this person, within a giant infinity symbol. A thread of pink light connects your hearts together. Imagine sending love along this thread to the other person, as you express forgiveness. Speak to them from the heart. Then seal them in a bubble of light and watch as it lifts into the air and flies away.

The infinity symbol is associated with love and balance; using it in a simple visualization that generates loving energy will help you let go of anger, forgive the other person and move on.

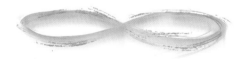

The Magician

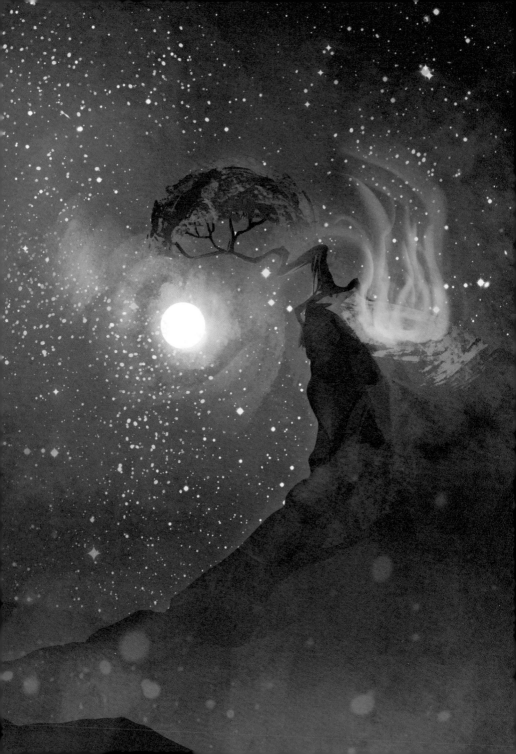

A GUIDED NARRATIVE TO:

Build inner strength

—

Step into your personal power

You are sitting at the top of a mountain. A blanket of stars rests above your head, and the night is rich with mystery. There's a light breeze brushing against your skin, and you feel expectant, as if something important is about to happen. You can see shapes in the distance, the outline of other mountains huddled together, and above them the full moon glows. You take a deep breath in and draw the cool air down into your lungs. As you exhale, you pour any fears into this outward breath. Peace permeates your being.

Sitting crossed legged, rooted to the spot, *you feel safe and secure*. From this vantage point you can see for miles around. Being so high up, so free, makes you feel in control and you take another deep breath, drinking in the power of this place. A tiny flame, a pinprick of light, sparks inside your belly, and it grows with every breath you take. The warmth spreads as the fire ignites, and you feel infused with strength. The moon turns her attention to you, bathing you in her luminescent stare. You smile, and *somewhere inside, at your very core, something solidifies*.

'I embrace my power,' you say.

Then, holding your hands out, you focus and hone your intent upon the space at your feet, as the fire within sizzles. A spark shoots from your fingers, igniting the ground in a cluster of flames. Where once there was nothing but dry earth, there now sits a small fire; a place to warm your soul. You are not surprised by this show of power. *You know you can do anything you set your mind to.*

Slowly rising, you turn, arms outstretched. You lift your face to the moon and spin, and as you do, the fire spreads in a perfect circle around you. This ring of flames provides protection and a sacred space where you can access your inner strength.

'I am strong,' you shout into the night.

As if in response, your words echo back.

'I am strong, strong, strong...'

Once more you sit in the centre of the circle you have created. The flames surge upwards, and the wall of fire cocoons you, making you feel even more empowered. It doesn't matter what lurks in the shadows, what lives upon the mountainside; this place is impenetrable. You place your hands flat upon the dusty terrain. A tingle vibrates in the middle of each palm, and then as you lift them upwards, a tiny sapling springs to life. It bursts from this brittle landscape pushing its head towards the stars, and you marvel at the new life you have created. The shoots twine around your fingers, and you feel earth energy mingle with your own essence.

It holds you firm.

Keeps you safe.

Defines your strength.

You take a gulp of refreshing air and feel your stomach swell. As you exhale, a stream of white light pours from your lips, it twists and turns until it forms a shape, a symbol to represent your personal power. The symbol hovers in the night sky above your head; a beacon of your strength for all the world to see. It shines as bright as the moon, and you know that whenever you need to feel emboldened, all you have to do is think of this symbol, bring it to the forefront of your mind and you will experience this energy again. *You can step into your power at any time.*

You watch as the symbol glides above the fire and then with a flick of your fingers, it becomes translucent, a heavenly waterfall dowsing the flames beneath. In seconds there is nothing left, the embers turned to ash and then completely absorbed.

Earth...

Air...

Fire...

Water

All the elements are at your disposal.

You are the magician, the master, the miracle.

The mountain draws around you and once more you are alone, peaceful and content. Streaks of charcoal line the sky and you marvel at their beauty. The inner warmth, the spark that sits at your core flickers brightly and *you know that you will always have the strength you need, in any situation, at any time.*

The earth supports you.

The elements are with you.

The power is yours.

'I am strong,' you call into the night one more time.

As the echo returns, a magnificent chorus that thunders between the mountain tops, you finally slip into a deep and restful slumber.

Affirmations

———

'The universe supports me in everything I do.'

'I am a magician, a master, a miracle.'

'Every breath I take, I am infused with strength.'

'I embrace my power.'

Boost your mindset

Continue to build a strong and fearless core with this exercise.

Think of the symbol from the story. If you don't have a clear image in mind, spend a few minutes pondering the word 'strength' and what it means to you. If you could choose a picture/pattern/image to represent strength, what would it be?

Allow some time to doodle and let your mind wander. When you have a symbol in mind, find a piece of paper and draw it. Trace over it several times until you are familiar with the shape and how it feels. As you do this repeat one of the suggested affirmations. Place the symbol somewhere you will see it every day, for example by your computer, on a fridge door/mirror etc. Whenever you see it, repeat the affirmation!

It's also helpful to draw smaller versions of the symbol on Post-it notes that you can position wherever you go.

A symbol can act as a trigger, so by choosing a symbol and an affirmation to represent a feeling, you immediately activate that feeling and step back into the story whenever you see it.

Journey to the Moon...

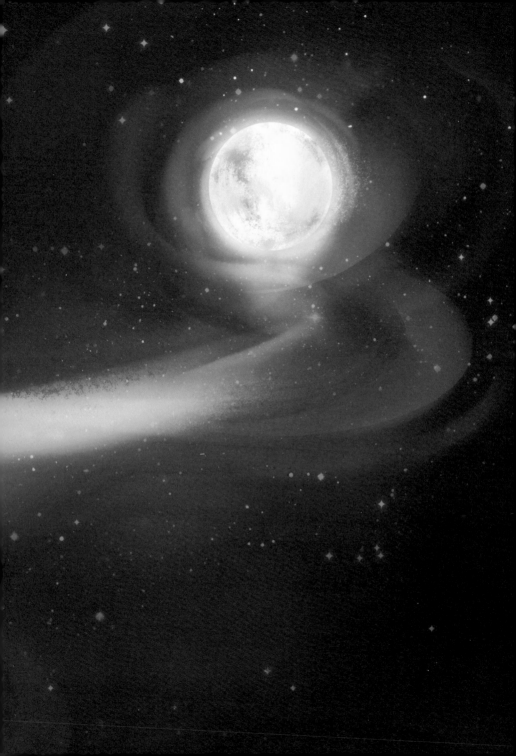

A GUIDED NARRATIVE TO:

Promote freedom

—

Help you seek out
new adventures

It is night and all the world's asleep. There's a hush, a pause in the pace of things. In the snug fit of the darkness of your room you feel safe, but excited too. Something is afoot. Something that will make your heart sing. You take a deep breath. Walk towards the window. The glass, a thin, transparent film, no longer feels like a barrier to the outside world. Instead it's an opening, a portal to somewhere new. The sky is host to thousands of stars. They glimmer against the velvet backdrop, and you're reminded of being backstage, the curtain shimmering ready to reveal you to your audience. A feeling of exhilaration fills your lungs.

It's your time and you are ready to step into the light.

You gaze up at the moon. Full and gleaming, this bauble of brightness takes your breath away. You wonder what it would be like to touch it, to be shrouded in luminescence. If only you could reach it with a click of your fingers, with a few magical words whispered into cobwebbed corners, then a rush of air and you'd find yourself soaring through time and space. But things like that only happen in stories.

A funnel of light catches your eye. It streaks across the sky and you wonder what it could be; a shooting star? It is sleek and graceful, swift and dipping like a murmuration of starlings. It's heading in your direction, picking up speed. As it gets closer, you see that it's a ball of white light. It blazes across the sky leaving a trail of glitter in its wake as it carves a path through the sky.

The shape gets closer and you feel that if you reached out your hand and the window wasn't there, you'd be touching. A million tiny pinpricks of light hold you in their gaze and you're lost for a moment in their beauty. The star emits a low hum. Warmth envelopes you and suddenly you are no longer behind the window. You are floating in the sky, cushioned by air – a being of light.

You want to ask, 'How is this possible?' but there is no time. You are flying, following in the wake of the shooting star. There is no need for words. No need for anything but the moment that you are in right now and you can't help but grin because *you are free*. In flight, in the heavens and with all of the universe to explore, *nothing is off limits to you now.*

Higher you climb, tailing your heavenly host. Clouds cluster at your feet, the earth is a tiny speck of dust and getting smaller with every breath. You are no longer tethered to one planet. *The universe is at your fingertips*. Ahead you see the moon, its waxen face lit with a silvery glow. Tendrils of mist spiral from the surface, like spectral hands they beckon you closer. The star hovers at your side and you know *this is your moment.*

Within seconds you are skimming the surface, feet touched by moondust. You feel each sole sink into white sand. The particles tingle against your skin and you feel alive, buzzing with energy. The air is sweet, and you drink it in, not bothering to wonder how you can breathe. Nothing is impossible in this time or place. Taking in the vista, you see a canvas of calm. The ground is a veil of white, and the air falls about you like a silk scarf. You walk, taking everything in. As you explore further you notice golden lights beneath your feet, darting in every direction like fireflies and you try to follow their path, until you become a part of the dance. Spinning, lunging, surging forwards; *you realize you are dancing on the moon.*

The ground is soft and spongy and with each footfall you bounce higher into the air. You are weightless, a being made of light, you sway and let the atmosphere cushion you. You spring from foot to foot and hoot with laughter as the lack of gravity lifts you up and away. All tension slips from your shoulders. The weight, both physical and emotional, dissolves as your spiritual energy takes on a waiflike form.

You look back upon the globe of the earth from your lunar vantage point and watch as it spins in the vast galaxy. The sheer enormity of life, the limitless vista that is your playground takes your breath way and you realize that you are one tiny being, one spark of light and you can go anywhere, and be anything. *Your imagination knows no bounds.*

You spin and weave, letting the universe support you while you explore this cosmic realm. Then finally, in a wave of content exhaustion, you collapse to the ground, letting the white sand of the moon become your mattress. Dust falls gently and blankets you, as you lie fully relaxed and full of promise.

Sleep beckons now, but tomorrow is a new day and *you can't wait for your next adventure!*

Affirmations

———

'This is my moment.'

'I relish the dance of life.'

'I am free to be what I want to be.'

'Ready for adventure, ready for *anything*!'

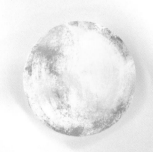

Boost your mindset

Expand your mind with this quick visualization.

Close your eyes and imagine your spirit slipping out of a hole at the top of your head. Your ethereal body expands, and you can feel your energy growing in every direction. Look around the space and see yourself from above, then expand further. Imagine your spirit body seeping through the walls that enclose you. Imagine it stretching in every direction. You can see for miles above and below and still you continue to grow, reaching up towards the sky and above the clouds. See the vastness of the universe and know that you are a part of this. You can go anywhere and be anything. There are no limits.

Say 'There are no limits' three times with feeling, then continue on with your day with a renewed sense of freedom!

The affirmation coupled with the mini visualization instantly takes you out of yourself and brings you into the current moment, while providing a vision of cosmic potential.

Acknowledgments

I'd like to say a massive thank you to my editor Chloe Murphy for her support, encouragement and inspiration. I'd like to thank the wonderful illustrator Alexandra for her beautiful artwork, which truly brings the words and ideas to life. I'd also like to thank the entire team at Quarto, and finally, a huge thank you goes out to my mum and dad, who knew the importance of a bedtime story to spark the imagination and ultimately soothe you to sleep.